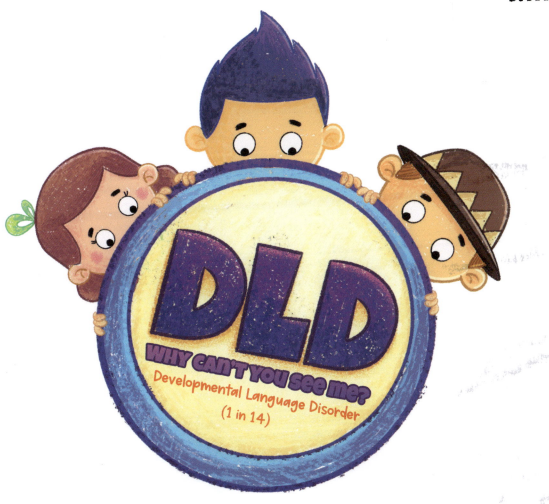

Written by
Shelbi Annison

I would like to dedicate this book to my family,
friends and to all the people who has supported me.
I would not be where I am today without you all!
To all the children, young people and adults with
DLD I want to see and hear from YOU!

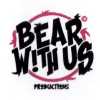

Published in association with
Bear With Us Productions

© 2022 Shelbi Annison
DLD Why Can't You See Me

The right of Shelbi Annison as the author of this work has been asserted by her in accordance with the Copyright Designs and Patents Act 1988.
All rights reserved, including the right of reproduction in whole or part in any form.

ISBN: 978-1-7395821-0-4

Design by Luisa Moschetti
Illustrated by Yogesh Mahajan

www.justbearwithus.com

Illustrated by
Yogesh Mahajan

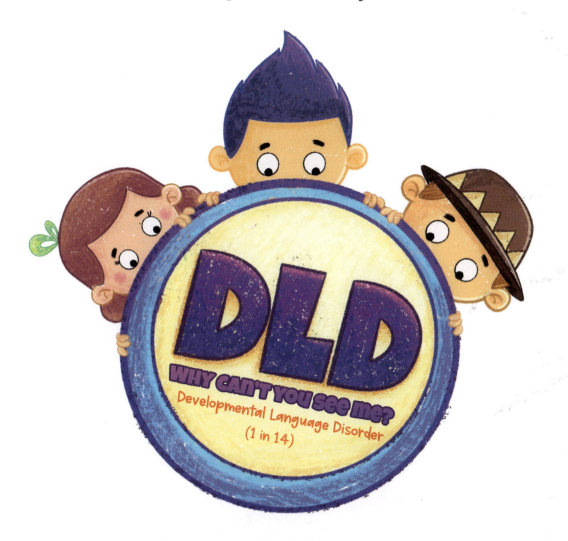

Written by
Shelbi Annison

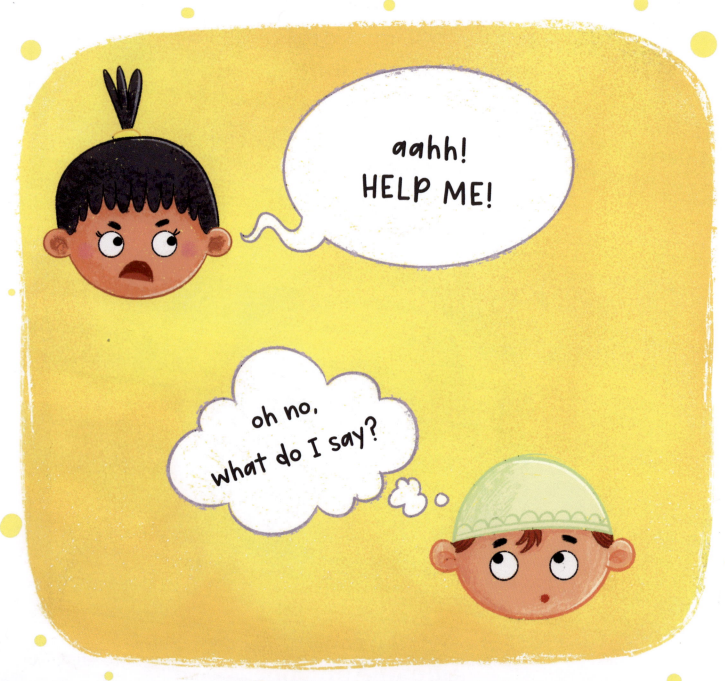

I might scream or shout; or freeze as no words come out

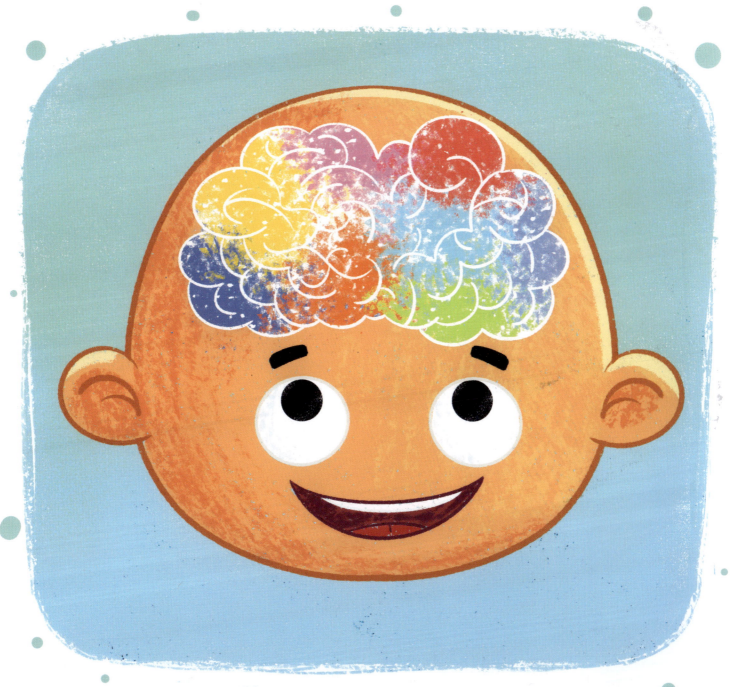

I might blend in or hide; wondering if I am different inside?

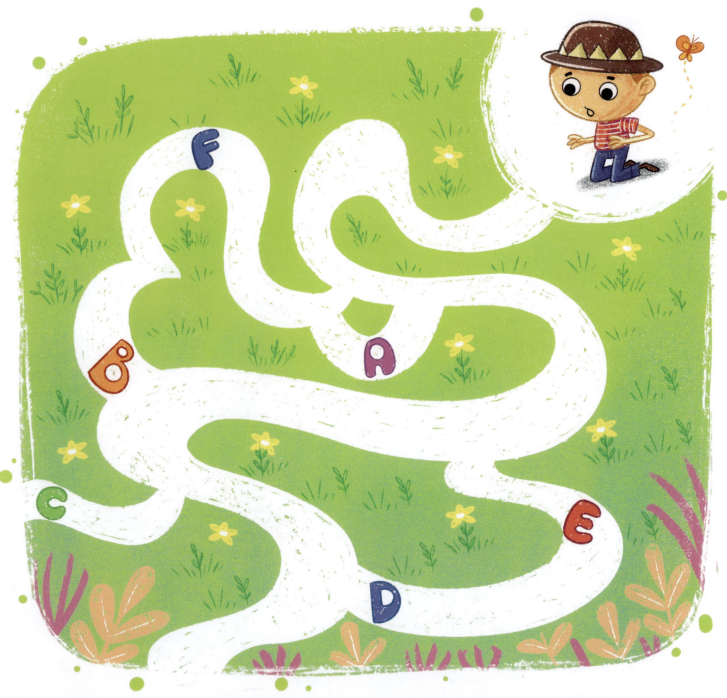

I might look or daze; fighting through the language is like a maze,

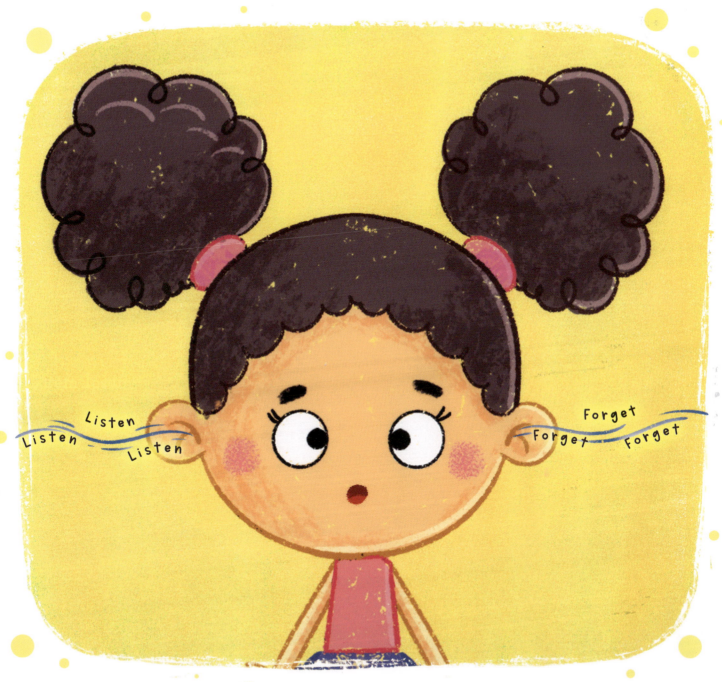

I might listen or forget; leaving me in a cold sweat,

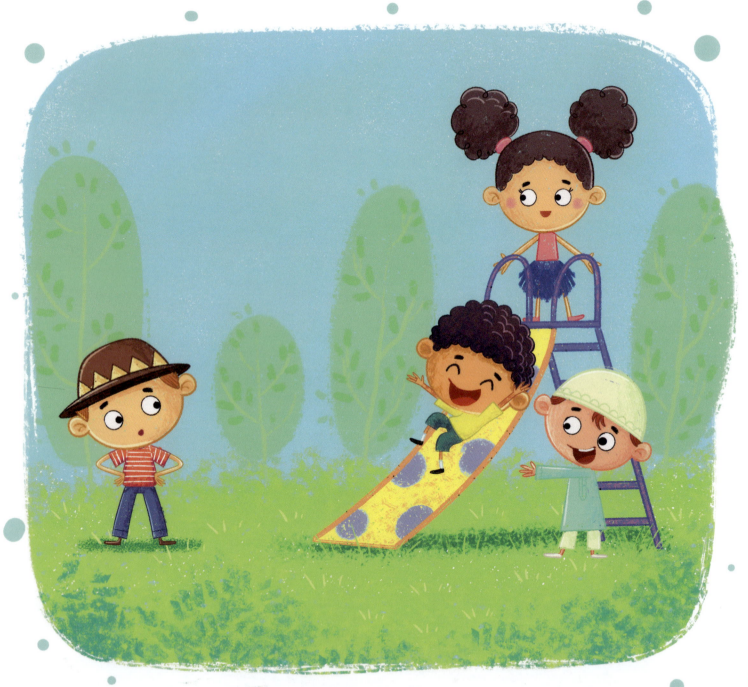

I might observe or play; wanting people to understand what I say,

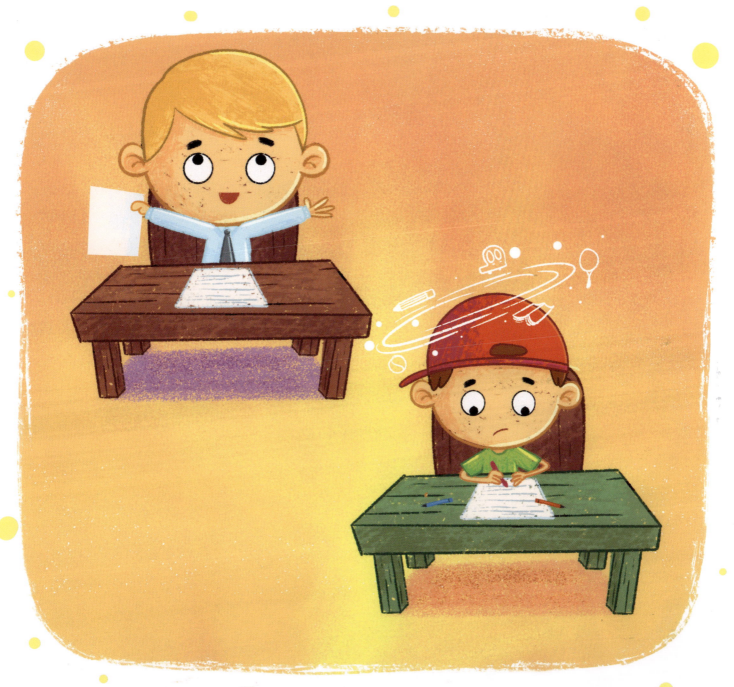

I might laugh or cry; you do not know how hard I actually try,

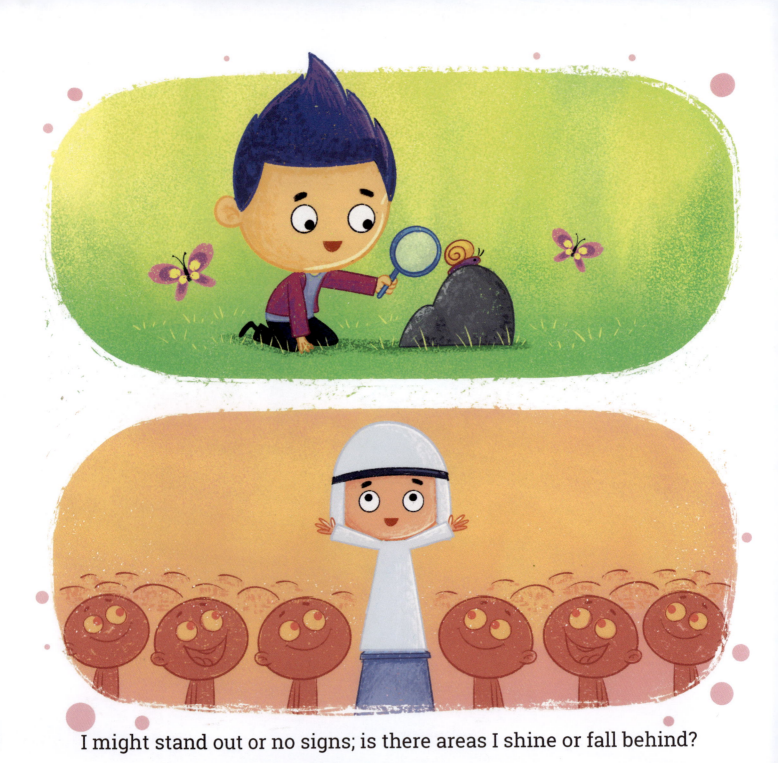

I might stand out or no signs; is there areas I shine or fall behind?

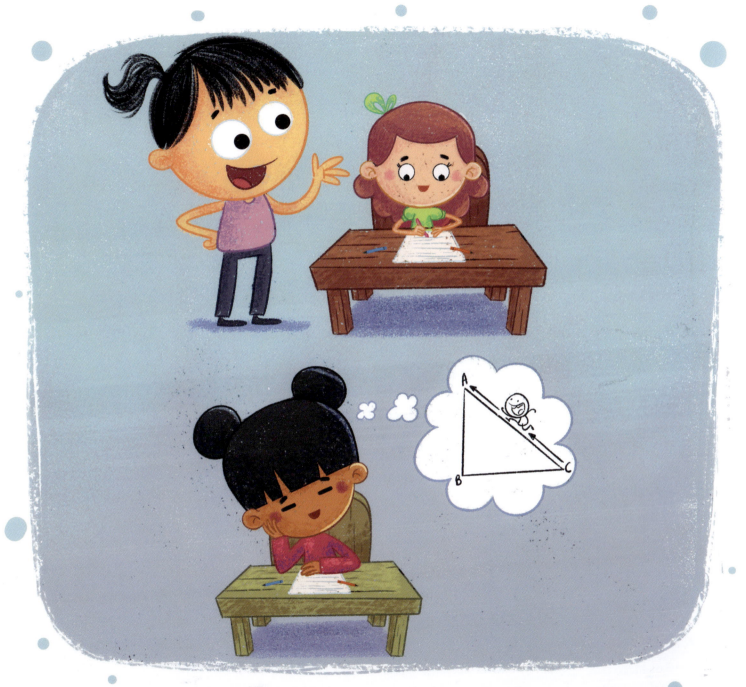

I might be alert or tired; exhausted, you do not know how much work is required,

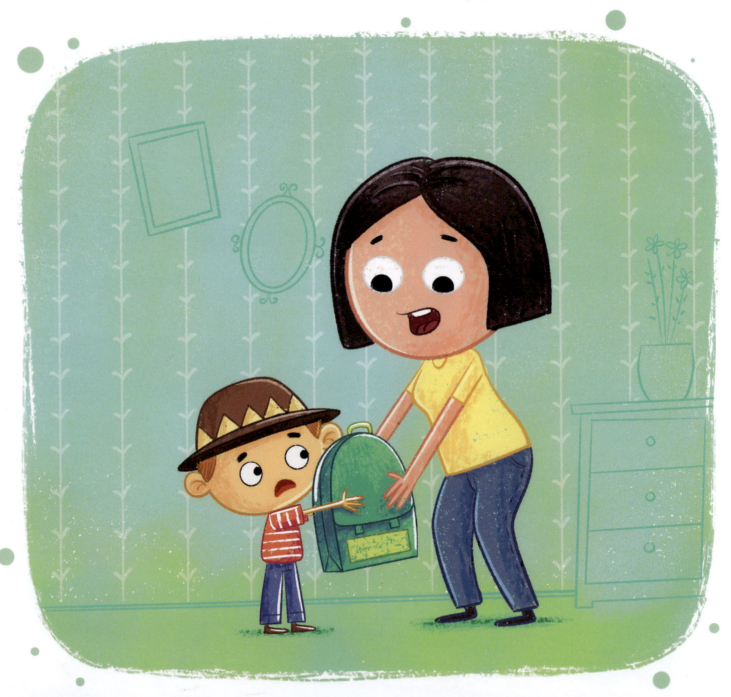

I might be quick or delay; processing and holding onto what you say,

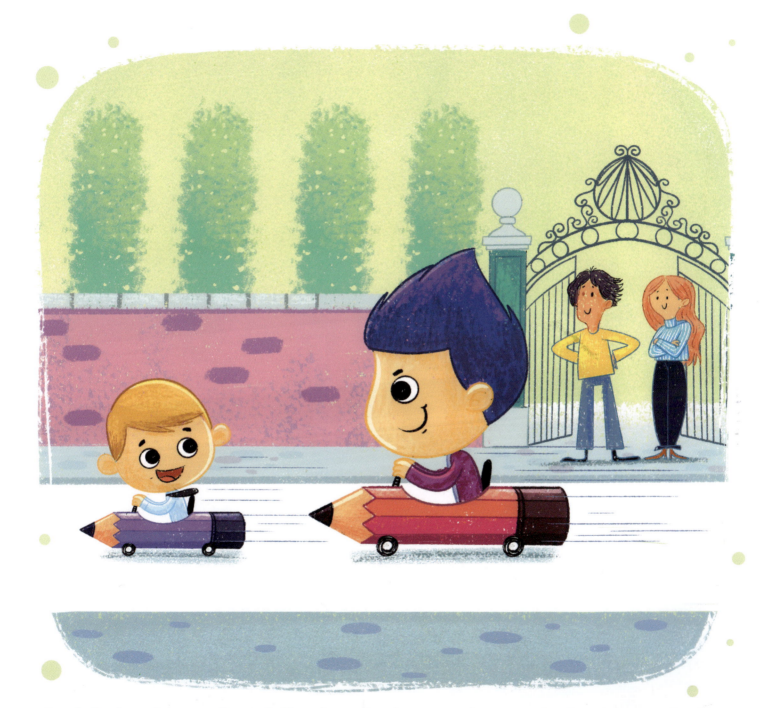

I might be slow or fast; following the instructions and what I am asked,

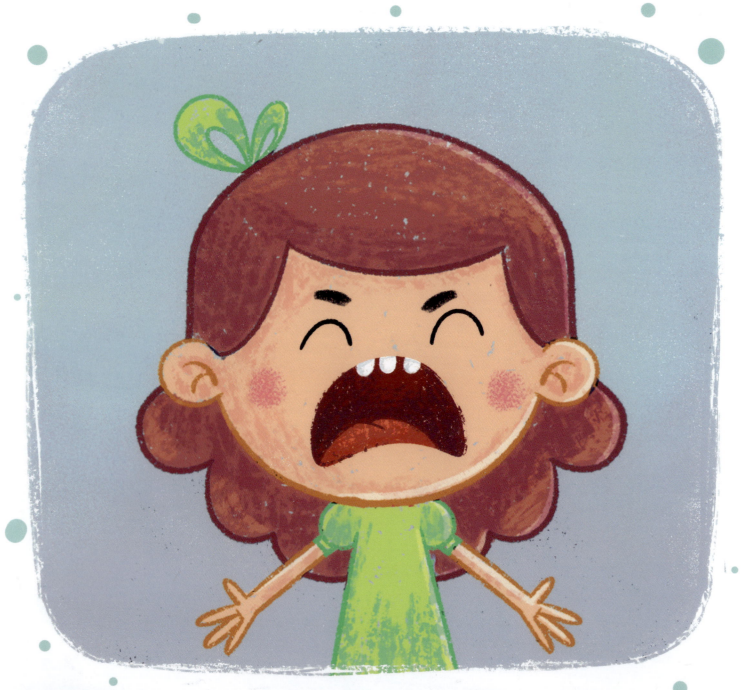

I might be hard-working or "lazy"; this misconception is driving me crazy,

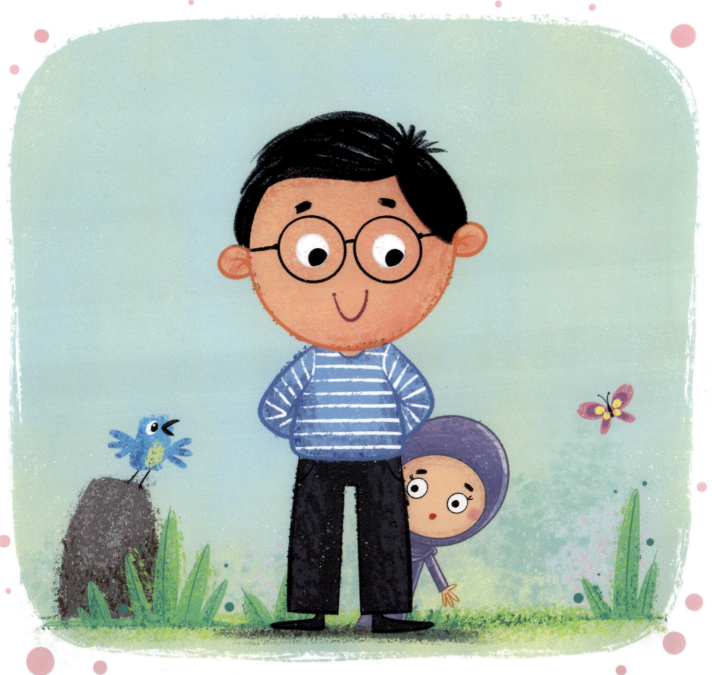

I might be loud or shy; sticking to somebody's side, scared of tongue tie

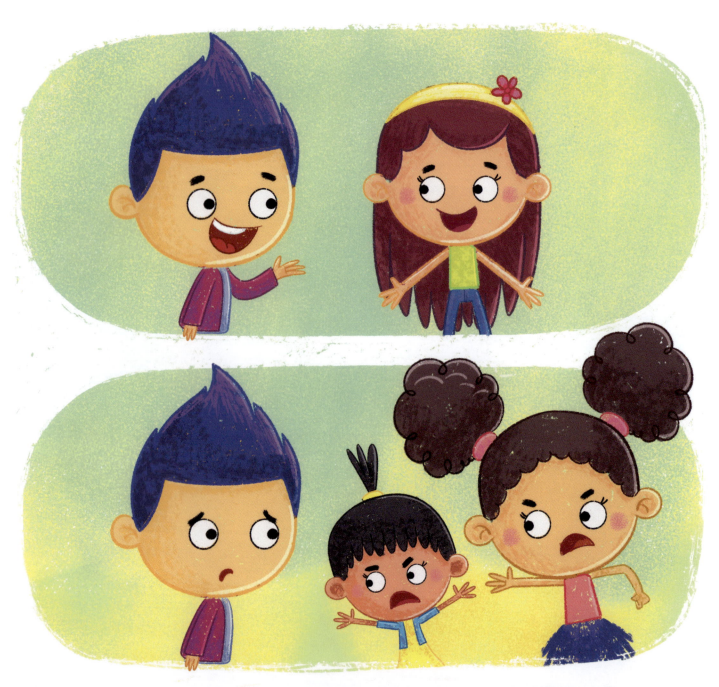

I might be nice or rude; without meaning to or having a clue,

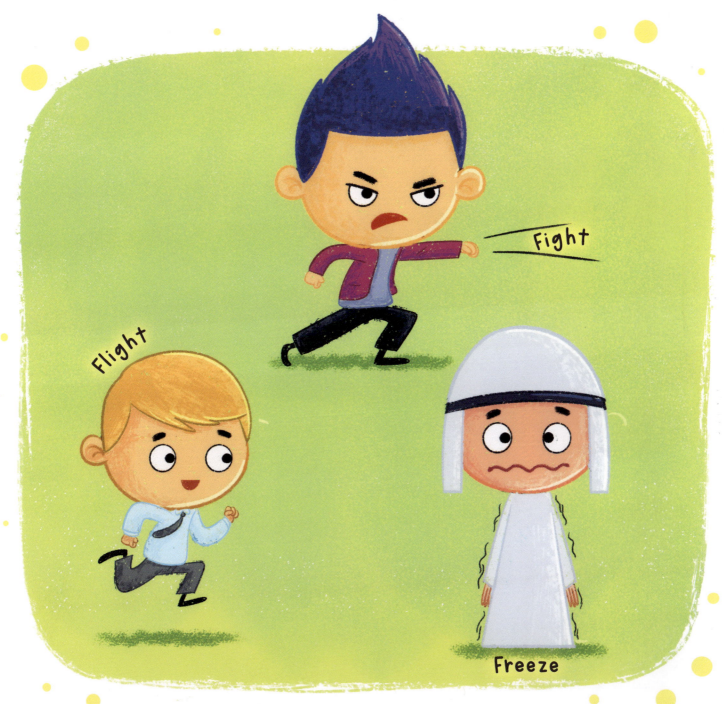

I might be high or low; expressing my thoughts and feelings, is hard to show,

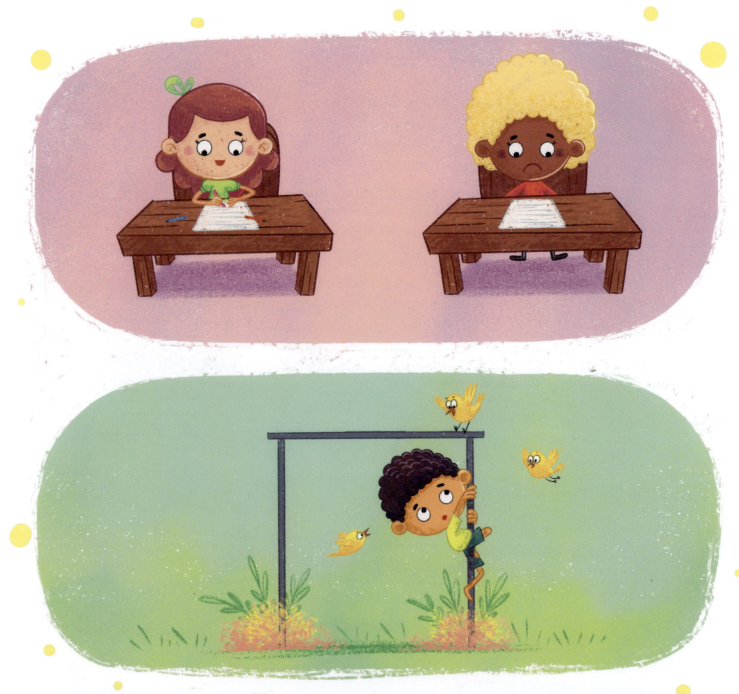

I might be good or trouble; but can you see how bad I struggle?

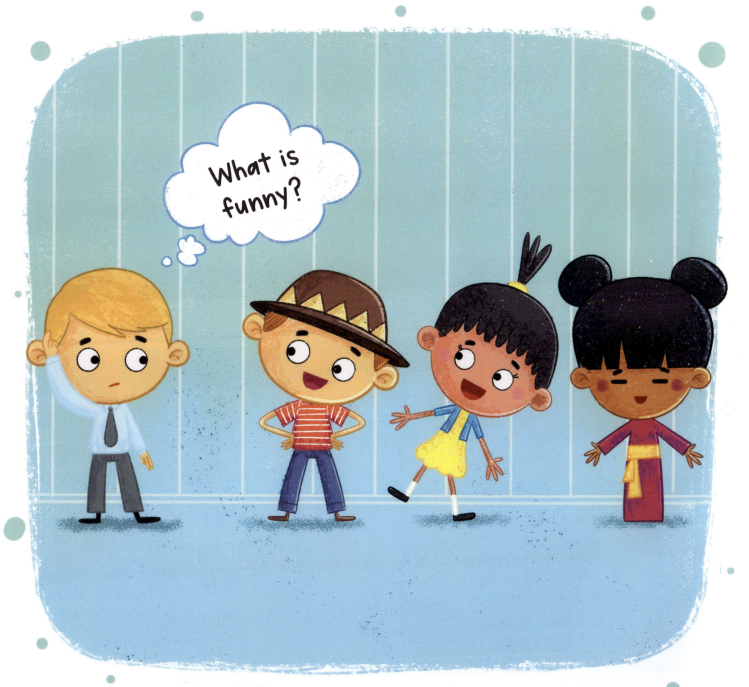

I might be serious or silly; what are jokes, idioms, and sarcasms? Really!

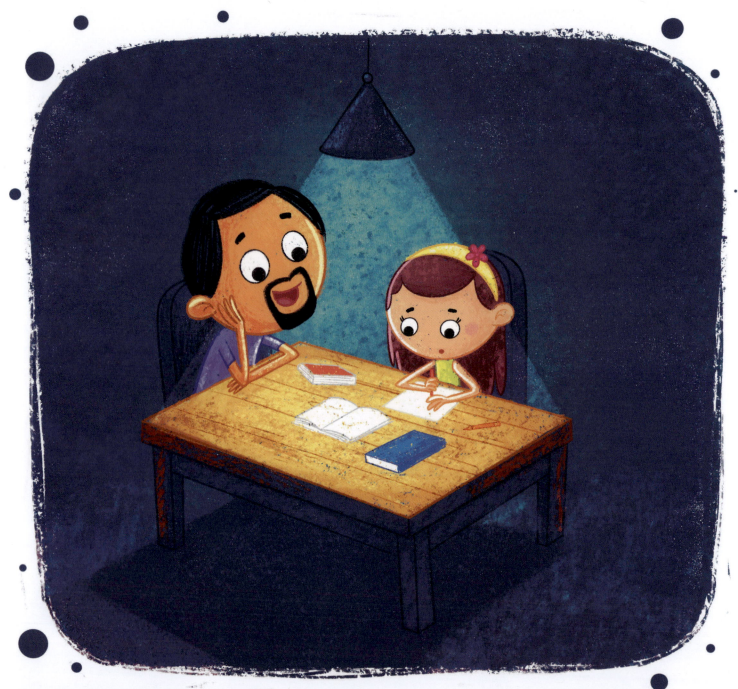

With support I can grow; the more I can show and will glow,

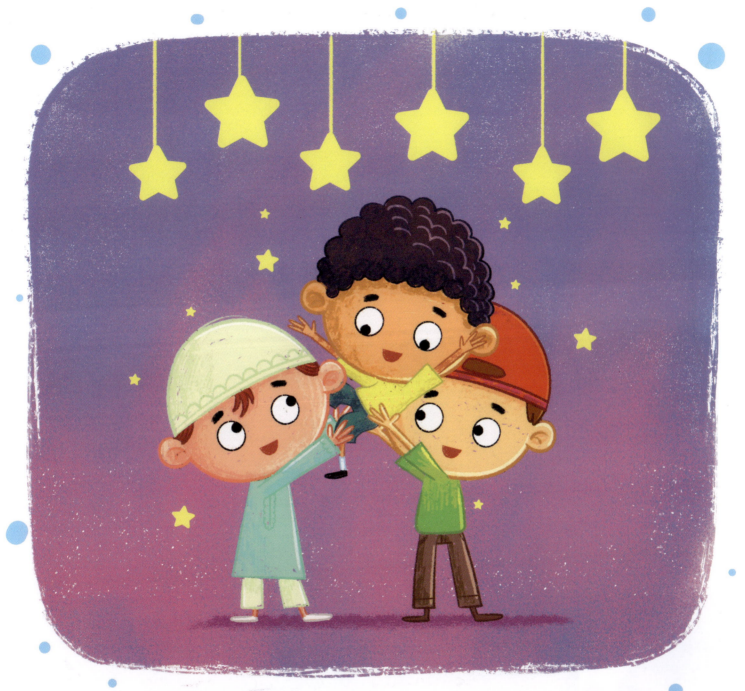

With support I can believe; the more I receive, I can achieve,

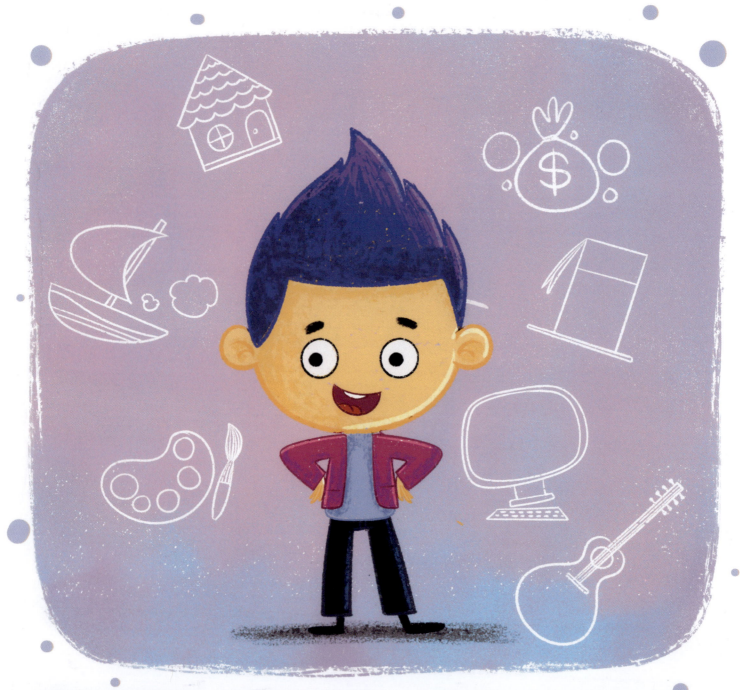

With support and confidence I gain; I can prove and show off my brain,

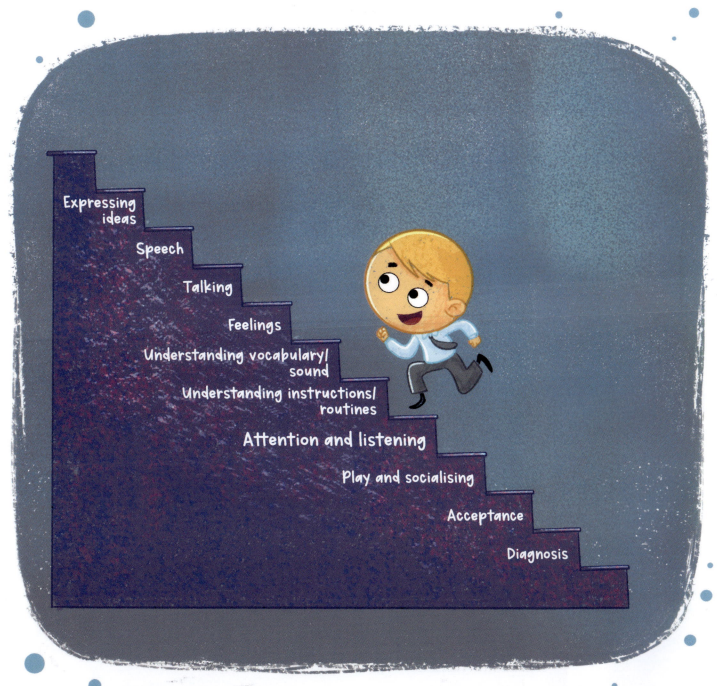

With support and extra time; the higher I can climb,

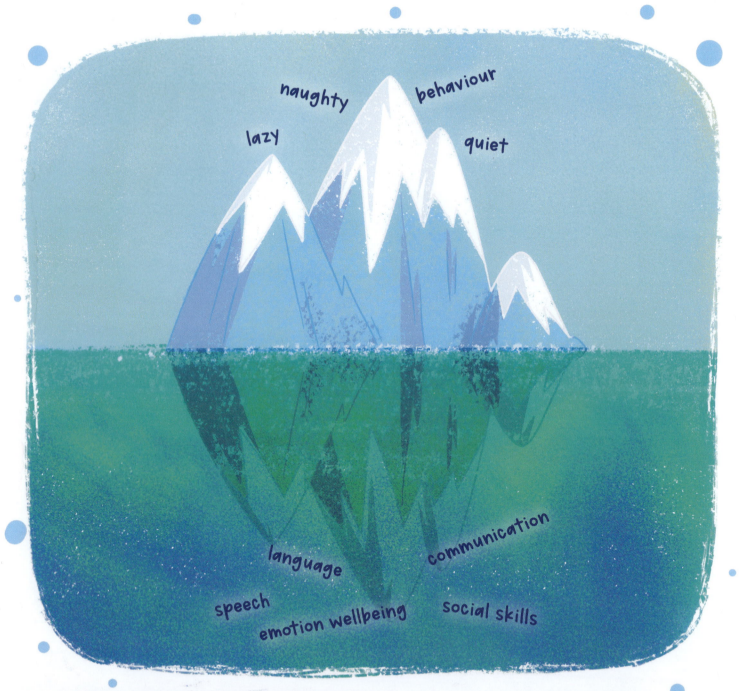

More than just "behaviour" you see; further unpicking is key,

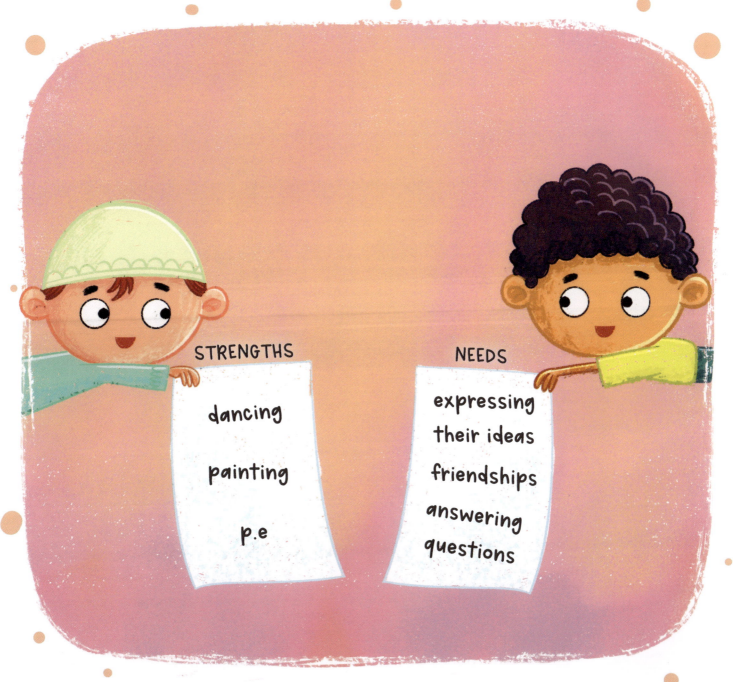

More than "ignoring"; the more I need exploring,

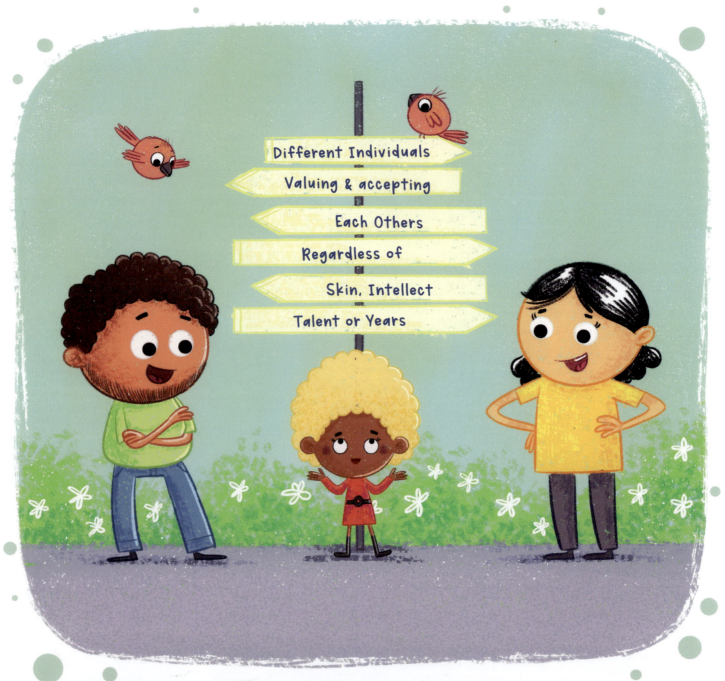

More than a "sad story"; listening and accepting is the glory,

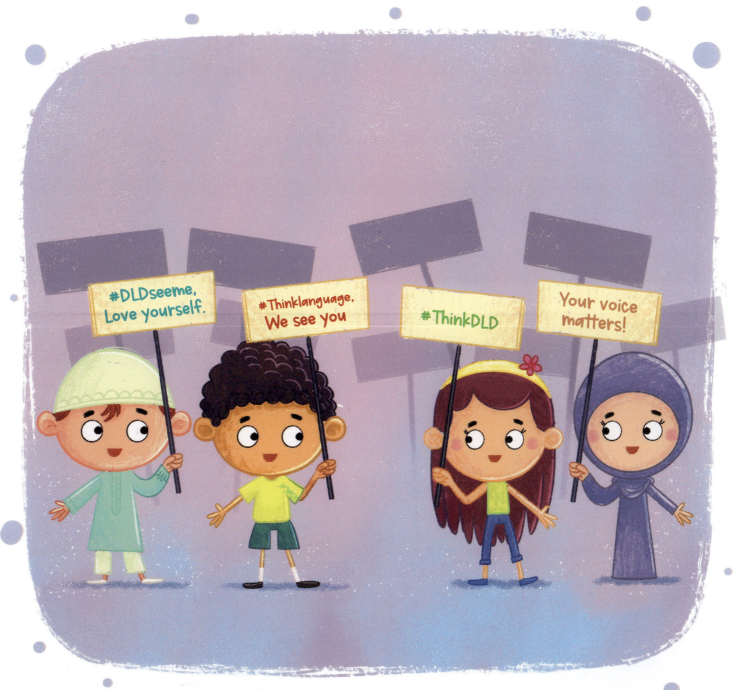

More than a "pain"; get on board with the #DLDseeme campaign,

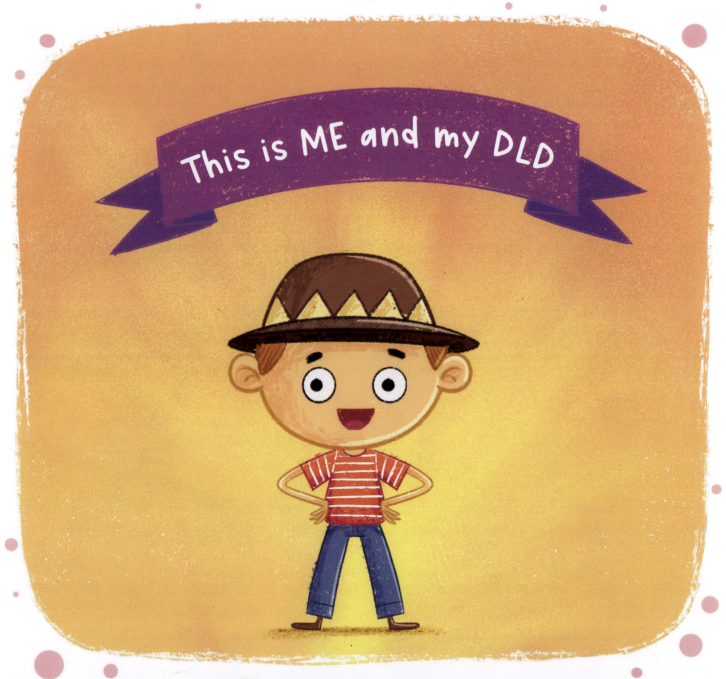

I have strengths and weakness; adding to my uniqueness,

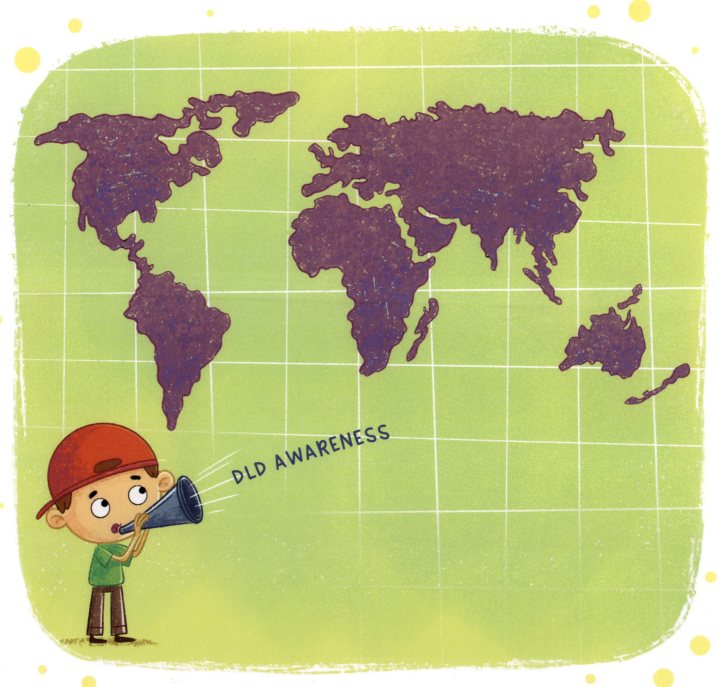

I have passion and ambition; raising awareness is my mission,

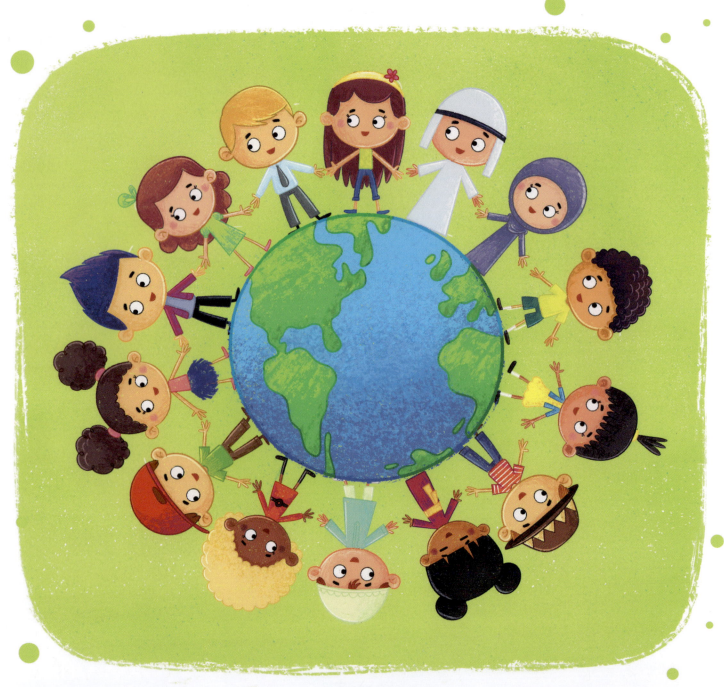

I AM MORE THAN A LABEL; I AM MORE THAN CAPABLE AND ABLE.

#DLDseeme

#Thinklanguage

#ThinkDLD

DLD; why can't you see me?!
About the Author

DLD; why can't you see me?! By Shelbi Annison, RADLD Ambassador

The inspiration behind writing this poem was after I received the diagnosis of Developmental Language Disorder as an adult – alongside my Dyslexia and short term memory. I wanted to help raise awareness of DLD, to try to explain the difficulties and impact that DLD can have, and to let other people with DLD to know you are not alone!

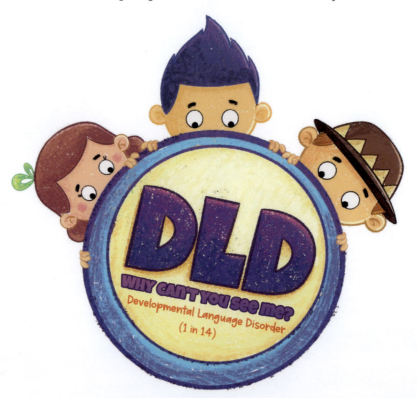

Further information and Support

- RADLD; RADLD | Raising Awareness of Developmental Language Disorder - **radld.org**
- AFASIC (UK) Afasic – Voice for Life - **afasic.org.uk**
- NAPLIC (UK) NAPLIC | NAPLIC - **naplic.org.uk**
- The DLD Project (Australia) The DLD Project | Information, Resources & Training - **thedldproject.com**
- Moor House School & College **moorhouseoxted.co.uk**
- DLD Tool Box Lisa Archibald(Canada) Language and Working Memory Lab - Western University - **uwo.ca**
- Ellen's DLD Website
- YouTube has amazing videos about DLD to explore!

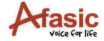 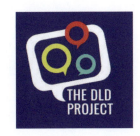 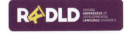

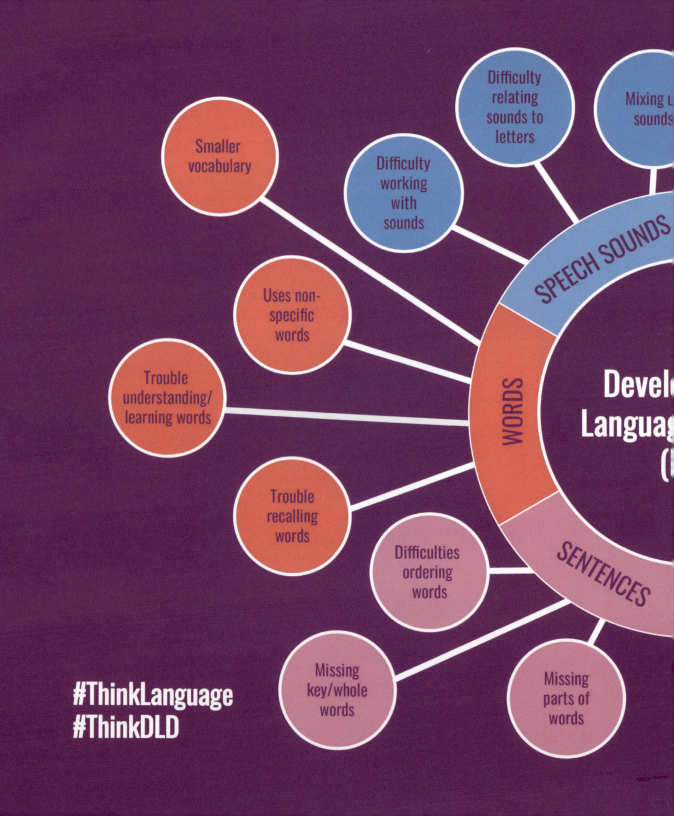

#ThinkLanguage
#ThinkDLD

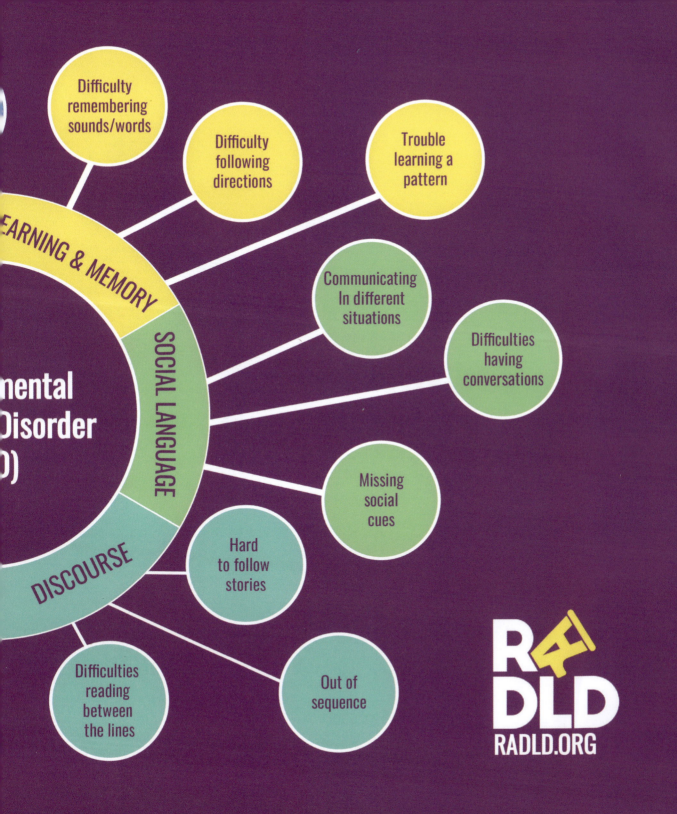

Printed in Poland
by Amazon Fulfillment
Poland Sp. z o.o., Wrocław